D1106031

ADPKD PATIENTS MANUAL

UNDERSTANDING AND LIVING WITH *AUTOSOMAL DOMINANT* POLYCYSTIC KIDNEY DISEASE

Irene T. Duley, RN, ANP
Patricia A. Gabow, MD

University of Colorado Health Sciences Center and Denver General Hospital

Polycystic Kidney Research Foundation
Kansas City, Missouri

National Institutes of Health Grant #5 P04 DK 34039

Printed in the United States of America by
The Polycystic Kidney Research Foundation

ISBN 0-9614567-4-4

Copy editors: Wendy Rueb, Deborah Hirsch

ACKNOWLEDGMENT: The Polycystic Kidney
Research Foundation wants to thank *THE
KIRKPATRICK FAMILY FUND* and *THE JEWISH
HERITAGE FOUNDATION OF GREATER KANSAS
CITY* for their contributions in support of this
educational publication.

Dedication

This booklet is dedicated to all the wonderful people who have participated in studies on Autosomal Dominant Polycystic Kidney Disease (ADPKD) at the University of Colorado Health Sciences Center since 1985 and to those of you who may do so in the future.

Thank you, all—You make a difference.

Foreward

Polycystic kidney disease research has come a long way. In 1985, the first major breakthrough occurred: the PKD gene was localized to chromosome 16. It took another nine years for the next big discovery: the ADPKD1 gene was identified in 1994.

In just the next **nine months** another major PKD research breakthrough occurred: the full sequencing of the PKD1 gene. The speed, frequency and magnitude of discoveries are increasing at an encouraging rate.

With research expanding so rapidly, our understanding of how PKD affects those who have it has increased, too. Much has been learned as to how PKD progresses and what treatment and cure opportunities lie ahead.

To help convey what we know about PKD, we are pleased to present this expanded and updated version of the PKR Foundation's **ADPKD Patients Manual: Understanding and Living with Autosomal Dominant Polycystic Kidney Disease.** We are exceedingly grateful to its authors, Irene Duley, RN, ANP, and Patricia A. Gabow, MD for their tireless efforts. We trust this resource will be enlightening to all who read it.

Finally, we are indebted to the countless PKD families we've come to know over the years. We are moved by your courage and resiliency and are grateful for the chance to serve your interests. Thank you for your example. To you and your loved ones, we commit ourselves and all our resources to discover a treatment and cure for polycystic kidney disease.

Dan Larson
President
PKR Foundation

Mission

The Polycystic Kidney Research Foundation is a 501(c)(3) not-for-profit public charity. It was founded in 1982 by Joseph H. Bruening. Its mission is to "promote research to determine the cause, improve clinical treatment and discover a cure for polycystic kidney disease" (PKD).

The PKR Foundation is the **only organization** worldwide that supports programs of research into the treatment and cure of PKD. In order to support this mission, the PKR Foundation fosters public awareness and education among medical professionals, patients and the general public.

Likewise, the foundation engages in extensive national efforts to develop funding for peer-approved biomedical research projects. It also works with the United States Congress to promote the importance of PKD research conducted by the National Institutes of Health.

For information about PKD or for assistance in becoming a member of the foundation, call or write the PKR Foundation at:

1-800-PKD-CURE　　4901 Main, Ste. 320
(1-800-753-2873)　　Kansas City, MO 64112
　　　　　　　　　　　　(FAX 816-931-8655)

Introduction to ADPKD

The purpose of this booklet is to provide information about Autosomal Dominant Polycystic Kidney Disease (ADPKD) to those who have the disease, those who are at risk due to an affected parent, interested family members and friends.

What is ADPKD?

ADPKD is an inherited disorder. It is passed from one generation to the next by an affected parent to a child. Although the primary manifestation of ADPKD is cysts in the kidney, cysts as well as other abnormalities can occur in other areas of the body. The other organs that can be involved are listed in Table 1.

How Common is ADPKD?

ADPKD has been estimated to occur in approximately 1:400 to 1:1,000 people of European descent. Although ADPKD has been seen throughout the world and among all racial and ethnic groups, it is not clear if the frequency is the same among all of these groups. For example, it has

Table 1

Manifestations of ADPKD in adults:

<u>Kidney</u>
Kidney cysts
Enlarged kidneys
Hypertension
Back and/or side pain
Blood in the urine
Kidney stones
Urinary tract infection
Kidney failure

<u>Cardiovascular</u>
Mitral valve prolapse
Aneurysm

<u>Gastrointestinal</u>
Liver cyst formation
Diverticula in the colon

<u>Other</u>
Cysts in other organs like the pancreas
  or spleen (uncommon)
Hernias

been said that ADPKD may be less frequent among American blacks than among whites.

How Does Inheritance Actually Work?

Our bodies are composed of billions of cells, all of which have two basic parts: the nucleus and the cytoplasm (figure 1). The nucleus is the control and operational center of the cell. It contains the message or blueprint inherited from our parents that determines what our cells actually do and what we will be like.

Each cell nucleus contains tiny threads called chromosomes. All the necessary information that is required to direct the formation and function of a human being is contained in these chromosomes. The chromosomes in turn are composed of genes, which are the basic units of heredity. Genes are so small that they remain invisible even under an electron microscope. Genes, therefore, are studied by molecular geneticists.

The building blocks of genes are chemical substances called nucleotides (figure 2). There are four nucleotides: adenosine, thymidine, cytosine and guanine, commonly expressed as **A**, **T**, **C** and **G**. Ultimately, everything in our body depends

3

figure 1

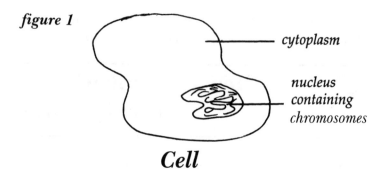

Cell

Our bodies are made up of millions of cells. Genes in the
chromosomes tell each cell exactly what to do.

4   *figure 2*

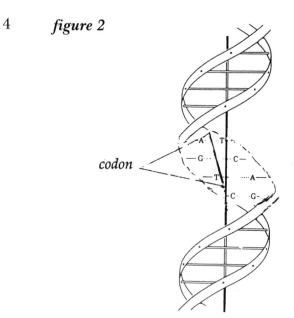

Deoxyribonucleic acid (DNA). A series of three nucleotides makes up one codon.

on how these four nucleotides are arranged. A sequence of three nucleotides is called a codon (figure 2). Genes are made up of codons. A small gene may contain 10 to 20 codons, whereas a large gene may contain many codons. Each codon codes for a certain amino acid. Thus, amino acids string together in a certain way to make a specific protein (figure 3).

Each protein has a unique function in the body. In a disease that is genetically inherited, there is some mistake or mutation in the gene. A single nucleotide change is enough to cause the gene to code for an abnormal protein that causes a disease. Therefore, the goal in ultimately curing a genetically inherited disease is to find out what the abnormal protein is and try to fix it.

What Do We Know About the ADPKD Gene?

An amazing thing we know is that there is more than one gene that causes ADPKD. There appears to be at least three genes that can cause ADPKD. About 80 percent to 85 percent of the people of European origin who have ADPKD, have the ADPKD gene located on chromosome 16, which is called ADPKD1. Most of the rest of the ADPKD population of European descent has the ADPKD gene located on chromosome 4 (figure 4); this is called ADPKD2. The location of the third gene has not as yet been determined. It is unknown which type of ADPKD genes are most common among other ethnic and racial groups.

It appears that the disease caused by the ADPKD1 and ADPKD2 genes are somewhat different. With the ADPKD1 gene, cysts seem to form at an earlier age, there appears to be an earlier onset of high blood pressure and earlier loss of kidney function as compared to the ADPKD2 gene.

Not only do we know where two of the ADPKD genes are located, but the nucleotide sequence of the ADPKD1 gene has been determined and some mutations identified.

How is ADPKD Inherited?

Every person has 23 pairs of chromosomes making a total of 46 (figure 4). Twenty-two pairs are called autosomes, and one pair determines the sex of an individual. Because the ADPKD genes are on an autosome, men and women have an equal chance of inheriting this disorder.

During reproduction, the chromosome pairs split in the formation of female eggs and male sperm. The woman donates 23 of her chromosomes to the baby in the egg and the man donates 23 in the sperm. In this way, when the egg is fertilized by the sperm, it will have the normal complement of chromosomes (figure 5).

figure 3

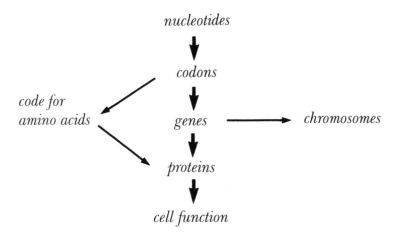

nucleotides

↓

codons

code for
amino acids

genes → chromosomes

↓

proteins

↓

cell function

7

Nucleotides are grouped to form codons; and codons are grouped to form genes. Each codon codes for a specific amino acid. The order of the codons determines the order in which the amino acids are grouped together to form a specific protein. Each protein in turn has a specific function in the body.

There are four possible ways the egg and the sperm of a couple in whom one has ADPKD can combine. Two of the possibilities will contain the chromosome with the gene for ADPKD and two will not (figure 6). Therefore, each child of a parent who has ADPKD has a 50 percent possibility of inheriting the affected chromosome.

If I have four children, does this mean that two of my children will have ADPKD and two will not? In real life it may not work out that two children will have the disease and two will not. The risk of having a child who inherits the chromosome with the affected gene is always 50 percent with each pregnancy no matter how many children a person has. It's like the flip of a coin: There is always a 50 percent chance of getting heads and a 50 percent chance of getting tails. In some families, all of the children are affected; in other families, none are. Many families with multiple children will have both affected and unaffected children.

In ADPKD there is also approximately a 6 percent to 10 percent rate of **spontaneous mutation**. This means that instead of inheriting the ADPKD gene from a parent with the disease, the gene mutates by itself for no known reason. That is, the sequence of nucleotides or codons resulting in ADPKD has permanently changed . It is important

figure 4

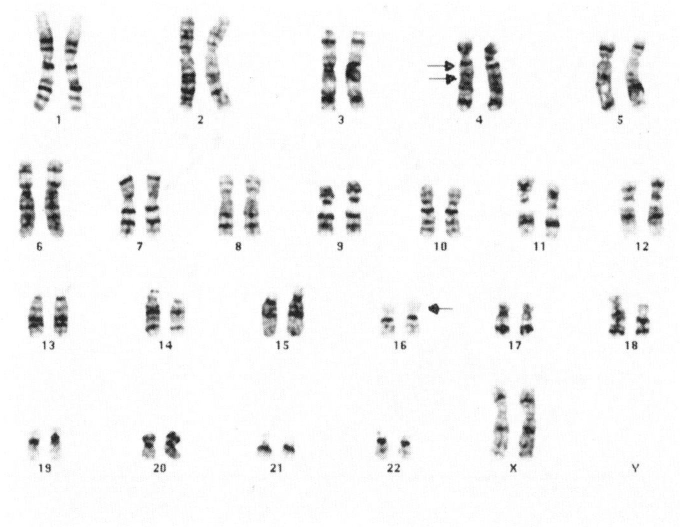

Example of the normal amount of chromosomes arranged in 23 pairs. Twenty-two pairs are called autosomes and one pair determines sex. This person is female and has two XX chromosomes and no Y chromosome. Chromosome 16 has the ADPKD1 gene on it and chromosome 4 has the ADPKD2 gene on it.

figure 5

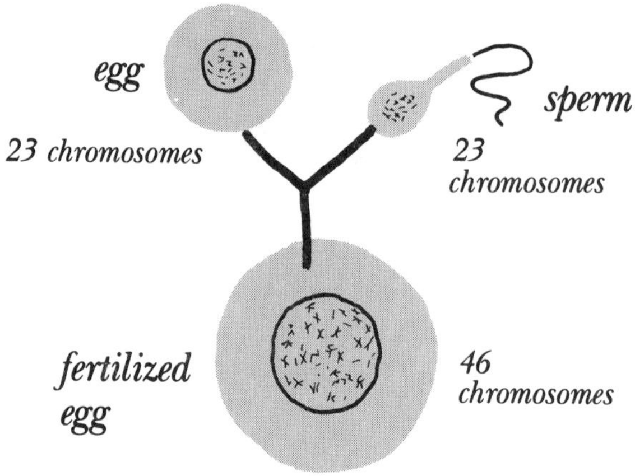

egg

23 chromosomes

sperm

23 chromosomes

fertilized
egg

46
chromosomes

Female egg with 23 chromosomes (1 of each pair), sperm with 23 chromosomes (1 of each pair) and fertilized egg with 46 chromosomes (2 of each pair).

figure 6

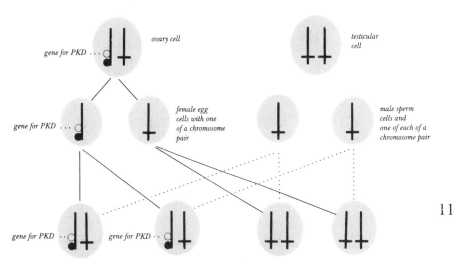

gene for PKD · · · ovary cell

testicular cell

gene for PKD · · · female egg cells with one of a chromosome pair

male sperm cells and one of each of a chromosome pair

gene for PKD · · · gene for PKD · ·

Example of how PKD is inherited:
Two female eggs, one with the gene for PKD and one without.
Two unaffected male sperms.
Four possible combinations of egg and sperm fertilization.
  The babies who inherit the PKD gene will have PKD. The babies
  who don't inherit the gene will not have PKD.

to know that even with a true spontaneous mutation, a newly affected person will still pass the
mutated gene on to his/her children.

Does Everyone Who Has the Gene for ADPKD Have the Disease?

The gene for ADPKD is dominant, which means
there only has to be one copy of the gene passed
on from either an affected mother or father to
cause the disease. There is *no carrier state* with a
dominant gene; it does not hide and come out in a
later generation. So if a person has the gene, at
some time in his/her life at least some of the manifestations of the disease will occur. When an individual does not have the gene for ADPKD, he/she
does not have the disease and therefore cannot
pass the gene on to the next generation.

However, that does not mean that everyone who
gets the ADPKD gene has the same signs or symptoms, the same age of onset or the same course of
the disease. In fact, there is a wide spectrum of
severity with ADPKD. At one end are children who
are diagnosed in utero or in the first year of life
with cysts and/or big kidneys, and at the other end
is the person who has few, if any, symptoms even
when quite old. Most people who have the ADPKD

gene fall in the middle and at some time will have some signs or symptoms associated with ADPKD.

Does Everyone Who is in the Same Family Have the Same Type of ADPKD?

Everyone in the same family has the same type of ADPKD gene and the same defect in that gene. However, even in the same family, signs and symptoms and the course of the disease are very often different. The most dramatic example of this occurs in families with children who are diagnosed in utero or in the first year of life. These children have signs of the disease long before their parent with adult-onset had signs. Often the parents of children who were diagnosed in utero don't even know they have the disease until after their child is diagnosed and they are subsequently tested.

Several ADPKD studies have recently been completed that look at how often kidney failure occurs at the same age in members of the same family. In one large study, almost half of the families had a member who progressed to kidney failure more than 10 years earlier than did his/her parent. Because of this, it is very difficult to predict the course of the disease in any one family member by looking at the progression of the disease in his/her parent or siblings.

How Does a Person Find Out if He/She Has ADPKD?

A physician is alerted to the possibility of ADPKD in three different settings: when someone reports that there is a family history of ADPKD, when there are signs and symptoms that commonly occur in ADPKD, or when a test is done for some other reason and cysts are found in the kidney.

Sixty percent to 70 percent of the time there is a family history of ADPKD. Family history helps to see who is at risk to develop cysts. In general, the signs and symptoms of ADPKD are not specific enough to permit a doctor to know if a person has the disease or not. For example, although some people with ADPKD have back pain and/or high blood pressure, so do many other people. However, if a person goes to the doctor with these signs or symptoms and the doctor also feels enlarged kidneys or liver during an examination, he/she will likely think about ADPKD and order an ultrasonogram.

Ultrasound is the best screening test for ADPKD. Ultrasound can detect cysts in nearly all people with the ADPKD gene who are over age 20. It does not use dyes or radiation and is relatively inexpensive. Rarely, ultrasonography will not be able to detect tiny cysts that can be seen with computed tomography (CT). The reason CT scans are not used as the first test to diagnose ADPKD is that CT uses radiation and often requires dye. CT scan is the best test when certain complications like bleeding into a cyst or kidney stones are suspected.

The limitations of both ultrasonography and CT scan is that the cysts have to be large enough to be seen. Early in the course of the disease, especially before age 10, a person can have one of the genes for ADPKD but not have cysts large enough to see. This is when a test for the gene is helpful.

In the future, a simple blood test may determine the ADPKD status of an individual. This is not yet possible; for now, gene linkage study is the most accurate test when the cysts cannot be seen by ultrasonography or CT scan. Gene linkage can determine ADPKD status with a 99 percent probability in informative families. However, gene linkage is quite expensive ($2,200/family) and requires several other family members with ADPKD to donate blood samples (figure 7). Because of this, gene linkage is usually used only when an undiagnosed family member would like to donate a kidney to another family member or when the outcome of a pregnancy would be altered if a positive diagnosis were made in the fetus.

figure 7

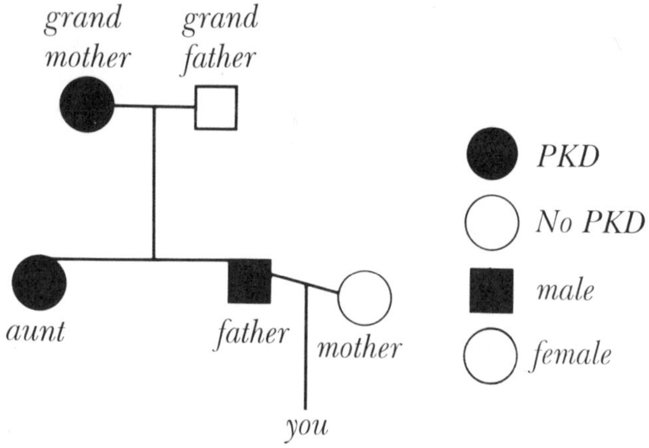

Example of an informative family for gene linkage analysis.

Since the Kidneys Are So Involved in ADPKD, What Should I Know About Them?

Each person is born with two kidneys, which are located in the back of the body on each side of the spine, tucked under the rib cage. The kidneys are about five-and-a-half inches long (14 cm), three inches wide (8 cm) and two inches thick (5 cm).

They weigh 10 to 12 ounces (figure 8). Both of the kidneys are affected when a person has ADPKD. There may be just a few cysts or many, and the cysts may range in size from a pinhead to the size of a grapefruit. If there are many cysts, the kidneys can more than double in size and weight.

Each kidney contains about 1 million tiny tubes called nephrons. A little over 22 percent of the blood the heart pumps every second goes to the kidneys. This blood flows through a filter (glomerulus) in the nephron (figure 9). Red blood cells, white blood cells and large substances like protein don't normally pass through the glomerulus but rather stay in the body. The fluid that goes through the filter is made up of water, electrolytes and other small substances.

About 150 quarts (158 liters) of fluid are filtered by the kidneys each day. The fluid passes through the glomerulus and the long tube of the nephron. All except 1-2 liters is reabsorbed back into the body; the rest ends up as urine. This process of filtering and reclaiming fluid along the nephron enables the normal kidney to maintain the body's fluid composition perfectly.

The kidneys are a regulating system. They make sure your electrolytes such as sodium, potassium, calcium, phosphorus and other chemicals are in balance. The kidneys also help regulate the pH of your body fluids so they are not too acidic or alkaline. The kidneys also filter and excrete waste products that your body produces each day.

---

figure 8

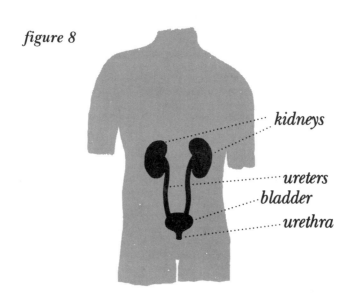

kidneys

ureters
bladder
urethra

Normal location of kidneys, ureters, bladder and urethra in abdomen.

Blood urea nitrogen (BUN) and creatinine are two waste products that are removed by the kidney. In particular, creatinine is removed so efficiently that an estimate of kidney function can be made by the level of this substance in the blood. Your doctor can calculate approximately how much actual kidney function you have with a blood test for creatinine, a 24-hour urine collection, and your height and weight. This is called creatinine clearance, glomerular filtration rate or GFR.

figure 9

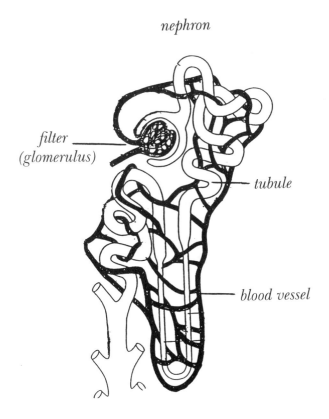

nephron

filter
(glomerulus)

tubule

blood vessel

The nephron (kidney tubule) is the functional unit of the kidney. Substances and fluid pass from the blood vessel into the tubule. There are about one million nephrons in each kidney.

Other functions of the kidney include making several essential hormones. One of these is renin, a hormone that in turn forms other hormones that help regulate blood pressure and the body's handling of salt.

Another hormone that is made in the kidneys is erythropoietin, commonly called EPO. EPO is a hormone that tells the bone marrow to make red blood cells. If a person's kidneys are surgically removed or if they fail because of a kidney disease, EPO is no longer produced and blood transfusions must be given to the person every five to seven weeks. The exact gene that codes for the protein erythropoietin was discovered several years ago. There is now a genetically manufactured form of EPO that a person can take, which eliminates the need for transfusions.

The kidneys also change vitamin D to its active form. In this way the kidneys help control calcium and bone formation. Because the kidneys perform all these functions, they are very important in keeping a person healthy.

What is a Cyst?

A cyst in the kidney begins as an outpouching of the nephron, similar to a blister. Cysts can occur anywhere on the length of the nephron. Although polycystic means many cysts, not every nephron forms cysts. The fluid inside the cysts often reflects the area in the nephron from which the cyst arose.

Approximately 70 percent of cysts detach from the nephron when they are still very small, about 2 mm (1/8 inch) in diameter. Over time the cysts enlarge and can become filled with clear fluid or fluid that contains blood or white blood cells.

Cysts can form in other organs as well as the kidney; the most common other site is the liver. Current research suggests that liver cysts are associated with the bile ducts or tubules of the liver rather than liver cells themselves. It appears that rather than take the place of functioning liver cells, cysts merely push the liver cells aside. This is why liver cysts don't cause liver failure even though the liver can become quite enlarged due to cysts.

What Causes Cysts to Form?

The gene that causes ADPKD gives an incorrect message and makes an abnormal protein. This causes some cells in the body to function incorrectly. As yet we don't know what the abnormal message or protein is, but we can see some of the abnormalities that result. For example, research has shown that there are at least three components to cyst formation (figure 10):

1. **Cell proliferation**. The cells of a cyst wall

reproduce themselves more than do normal kidney cells. This makes the cysts grow in size.

2. **Cellular secretion.** Secretion is a way of making fluid. To form a cyst the cells themselves must produce fluid. If there were no fluid produced to fill the cyst, there would merely be a ball of cells.

3. **Abnormal basement membrane**. The basement membrane is a very thin layer of tissue the cyst cells sit on. In ADPKD this layer is thicker than usual and is made up incorrectly.

Research is continuing on other complex factors that affect cyst formation and growth.

How Do Cysts Cause Problems?

In general, cysts cause problems because of their size and the space they occupy. Many of the symptoms people with ADPKD have depend on how big their kidneys and liver are. The size of the kidneys and liver is directly related to how many and how big the cysts are. For example, people with kidneys over 15 cm (6 inches) are more likely to have pain than people with smaller kidneys; people with ADPKD who have high blood pressure have bigger kidneys than those with normal blood pressure; people with ADPKD who have bleeding into their urine have bigger kidneys than those who don't;

and, individuals who have large kidneys have more loss of renal function than people with smaller kidneys.

Normal tubule with a normal basement membrane

small cyst with thick basement membrane and more cells

figure 10

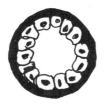

Cyst with thick basement membrane and increasing number of cells containing an increased amount of fluid

Example of cyst formation

How Will I Feel if I Have ADPKD?

Early in the disease there generally are no symptoms at all. In fact, many people are never diagnosed with ADPKD because they have so few or no symptoms. Often the first sign is high blood pressure, blood in the urine or a feeling of heaviness/pain in the back, sides or abdomen. Sometimes the first sign is urinary tract infection and/or kidney stones.

Can You Tell Me More About the Signs and Symptoms of ADPKD?

HIGH BLOOD PRESSURE

High blood pressure, or hypertension, affects about 60 percent to 70 percent of people with ADPKD. High blood pressure begins early in the course of ADPKD. Fifty percent of people with ADPKD who have normal kidney function already have hypertension. Twenty percent to 30 percent of children with ADPKD also have hypertension. Many times the increase in blood pressure will be the first sign of ADPKD and the reason a person gets tested. Hypertension occurs more commonly in men than in women. People with high blood pressure and ADPKD have more and larger cysts than do people with normal blood pressure.

Blood pressure is a measurement of the force the blood has as it flows through the body. This pressure depends on the amount of blood and fluid in the body, how much blood the heart pumps each second (called cardiac output), and to what degree the blood vessels are constricted or dilated.

It is similar to the force it takes to get water through a garden hose. The pressure depends on how much water is going through the faucet and how narrow the hose is.

Blood pressure measurements have two parts, which are recorded as millimeters of mercury (mm Hg), for example, 120/80 mm Hg. The top number or systolic blood pressure measures the pressure when the heart is actually pumping. The bottom number or diastolic pressure is a measurement of the pressure when the heart is relaxing between beats.

A great deal of research has been done trying to understand how hypertension occurs. In general there is either an increase in cardiac output or constriction of the blood vessels. In ADPKD it seems that the most likely of these two processes is the constricting of blood vessels. This is most often caused by one of a group of hormones.

As mentioned previously, renin is a hormone that is produced in the kidney. Renin acts on angiotensinogen, a substance in the blood that forms another hormone called angiotensin. Angiotensin is a powerful constrictor of blood vessels.

In ordinary circumstances the kidneys make renin when the blood pressure is low and the kidneys sense that they need a stronger flow of blood; so it is basically a protective mechanism.

In ADPKD, cysts can press on blood vessels in the

kidney (figure 11), resulting in decreased blood flow to some parts of the kidney. Sensors in the nephron react as though the blood pressure in the kidney was low; renin is then secreted, which in turn generates angiotensin, constricting the blood vessels, and causing high blood pressure.

figure 11

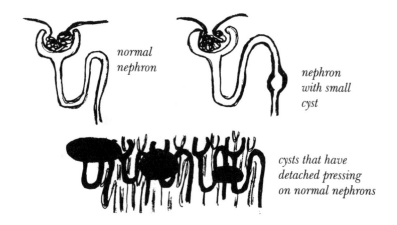

normal nephron

nephron with small cyst

cysts that have detached pressing on normal nephrons

Nephron with no cyst, nephron with small cyst, and nephrons with many cysts.

Whatever the initial cause of high blood pressure, it needs to be treated. If not treated, hypertension damages the kidneys, enlarges the heart and can cause strokes.

Hypertension in ADPKD is often treated by a group of drugs called angiotensin converting enzyme inhibitors (ACE inhibitors). This class of drugs is commonly used because of the role of angiotensin in causing high blood pressure in ADPKD. In general, ACE inhibitors are both safe and effective, but in some patients with large kidneys and decreased kidney function ACE inhibitors can make kidney function worse.

Regardless of what kind of blood pressure medicine is used, the most important thing is to have your blood pressure in or near the normal range. There are many different, very good medications to treat high blood pressure. Work with your doctor to find the right one for you. Remember, a blood pressure medicine only works if you take it! So try to have a regular time to take your medicine so that you don't forget.

Although drugs are important in treating blood pressure, in some individuals certain nondrug treatments also lower blood pressure. Some of these nondrug therapies include weight loss, exercise, low salt and a high potassium diet.

These treatments have not been studied specifically in ADPKD patients, but they are worth trying since they also improve a person's overall health.

WEIGHT LOSS   Weight loss in some people who are overweight can lower or eliminate the need for blood pressure medications.

EXERCISE	In some people regular exercise can decrease blood pressure. In everyone, exercise improves muscle strength and heart function.
ALCOHOL	People who drink more than three ounces of alcohol a day tend to have higher blood pressures than those who are nondrinkers or light drinkers.
SALT	Even though salt intake has not been shown to be the cause of hypertension in ADPKD, a low salt diet may be helpful, particularly if certain drugs are being used.
POTASSIUM	Although it has not been examined in ADPKD, in other causes of hypertension potassium can lower blood pressure. Interestingly, tests done on people who did not have ADPKD showed that low potassium actually caused cysts to form. It is unknown at this time if low potassium causes worsening of cysts in ADPKD. Therefore, a diet

28

that is high in potassium is probably a good idea (see diet) **if your kidney function is in the normal range.**

Discuss a high potassium diet with your physician to make certain that your kidney function is in the normal range. When kidneys start to fail they can't excrete the potassium properly, which could cause serious problems.

TOBACCO

Smoking increases the risk of heart disease and stroke. Smoking paired with hypertension increases these risks.

The large National Institutes of Health study, Modification of Diet in Renal Disease (MDRD), did not show any improvement in kidney function in ADPKD subjects whose blood pressure was strictly controlled. However, the people who participated in the study already had a considerable loss of kidney function. And the study was for only two years. Given the other effects of high blood pressure on the heart and brain, it is still important to control the blood pressure. At this time, we do not know what the best blood pressure level is for a person with ADPKD. However, some studies have shown the association between high blood pressure and progressive loss of kidney function with ADPKD.

If you have ADPKD you should have your own blood pressure cuff and monitor and keep a log of blood pressures away from the doctor's office. This will give your physician a better representation of your blood pressure over time.

Pain

Pain can be acute, signaling a sudden new problem like bleeding into a cyst, infection, or a kidney stone. Pain can also be a lingering problem, and then it is described as chronic.

Chronic pain is one of the most common problems for people with ADPKD. The pain is usually in the back or the side and occasionally in the stomach. The pain can be intermittent and mild requiring only occasional mild pain medicine such as acetaminophen. In a small number of people, the pain can be constant and quite severe. For these few people, cyst decompression can be very helpful. If there are a few big cysts that seem to be causing the problem, they can be decompressed. This is done by using ultrasonography and inserting a needle into the cysts, draining the fluid and coating the cyst wall with alcohol so the cyst doesn't make more fluid. If there are a great many small cysts causing the problem, surgical decompression can be done. Pain is a very subjective feeling. There is no way pain can be measured except by the person who is experiencing it. It is important to remember that pain frequency and tolerance vary greatly among individuals. Pain tolerance appears to be influenced by a person's cultural background, expectations, behaviors, and physical and emotional health. For this reason pain clinics that utilize biofeedback and support groups can also be very helpful to some people.

Blood in the Urine

Close to 50 percent of those with ADPKD have had or will have blood in their urine at some time. This is called hematuria. The urine may look pink, red or brown. Passing small amounts of red blood cells in the urine that can only be seen under a microscope may also occur. This is called microscopic hematuria.

Hematuria is more common in an individual with large kidneys and high blood pressure. It is thought that the rupture of cysts or small blood vessels around them is the cause of blood in the urine. Kidney and bladder infections and kidney stones can also cause blood in the urine.

Blood in the urine can last for a day or less or the bleeding may go on for days. Notify your physician if you see blood in the urine. Strict bed rest, increased fluid intake, and acetaminophen (if there is pain) are usually the treatments if the bleeding is prolonged. Avoid taking nonsteroidal anti-inflammatory medications such as aspirin or ibuprofen as they may prolong the bleeding. If bleeding is directly into a cyst, there may not be blood in the urine but pain can be severe.

An association between multiple episodes of hematuria and decreasing kidney function has been made. Therefore, if a particular activity is generally associated with blood in the urine, it would be best to avoid that activity.

Urinary Tract Infection

Urinary tract infection, commonly called UTI, is an infection caused by bacteria that have reached the bladder, kidneys or the cysts themselves. Other names used for UTI are cystitis for bladder infection and pyelonephritis for when the infection is in the kidney but not in a cyst.

The infection usually starts in the bladder and can progress up the ureters into the kidneys. Although both men and women have UTIs, they are far more common in women. This is due to women having a very short urethra (the tube that goes from the bladder to the outside).

UTIs are quite common in the general population, but they may be more frequent in those with ADPKD. Both males and females with ADPKD may be more likely to have an infection after a catheter is placed into the bladder. There seems to be an association between UTI and worsening kidney function in men but not in women with ADPKD.

The most common symptom of UTI, particularly if the infection is in the bladder, is pain or burning with urination and/or an urgent need to urinate even though there is only a small amount of urine passed. When the infection is in the kidney or in a cyst, there may be a sudden onset of fever, chills and back or flank pain.

Your physician should be notified if any of these symptoms occur so that treatment can be started. Usually a urine sample will be taken for a culture to see what kind of bacteria is causing the infection, and the appropriate antibiotic can be prescribed.

Women who have frequent bladder infections may decrease or eliminate the incidence by:

- ◆ Wiping from front to back after urinating or a bowel movement. This prevents dragging bacteria from the anus and vagina to the urethral opening.

- ◆ Drinking fluid prior to intercourse and

urinating afterward. This may help flush out any bacteria that may have entered the urethra.

- For those who have many UTIs, antibiotics may be prescribed on a daily basis to prevent recurring infections.

Kidney Stones

Kidney stones occur in about 20 percent to 30 percent of people who have ADPKD compared to 8 percent to 10 percent in the general population. One reason kidney stones are more common may be due to cysts blocking the tubules, preventing normal drainage. When the urine stays in one area longer than it should, crystals can form and cause kidney stones. Uric acid and calcium oxalate are the two most common types of crystals that lead to stones.

Another reason that stones may form in some people with ADPKD is that there is a decrease in urine citrate. Urine citrate is a substance that prevents formation of kidney stones.

The symptoms of kidney stones are severe pain in the back, side or into the groin. Often there will be blood in the urine when passing a kidney stone.

Kidney stones are treated the same way they would be if a person did not have ADPKD. Sometimes a machine that uses sound waves, called a lithotriptor, may be used to break the stones into smaller pieces so they can be passed.

Does Everyone with ADPKD Eventually Need to Have Dialysis or a Transplant?

Although everyone with the ADPKD gene develops kidney cysts, not everyone progresses to kidney failure, and if they do it's rarely before age 40. Several recent large studies have shown that about 70 percent of those with ADPKD have not progressed to kidney failure by age 50. These studies also showed that about 50 percent were not in kidney failure even at age 60, and 23 percent were not by age 70. There is a high probability that many people with a very mild form of ADPKD are unaware of their status and are never diagnosed.

Although we still don't know exactly how kidney failure happens in ADPKD, we do know some of the factors that increase the rate of progression to kidney failure. These include:

> Having the ADPKD1 gene as opposed to the ADPKD2 gene.
> Being male.
> Being diagnosed with cysts at a young age.
> Having high blood pressure.
> Having large kidneys.

Having many episodes of blood in
the urine.
Having urinary tract infections in men.
Being black.
Being black and having sickle cell trait.
Being a woman with high blood pressure
and four or more pregnancies.

Are There Other Problems Associated with ADPKD?

ADPKD is not just a kidney disorder; other organs can be affected (table 1). The list that follows may look long and overwhelming, but it's important to remember that most people don't have all of these problems. If you have ADPKD, you and your family should be aware of the following possibilities so you can play a major role in your own care.

Liver Cysts

Sixty percent to 70 percent of people with ADPKD have cysts in the liver during their lifetime. Liver cysts rarely occur in those under the age of 30 but do form and increase as a person ages.

The liver can remain normal in size with few cysts or become enlarged. Even though there is an increase in liver size, the amount of functional liver tissue remains fairly constant. Therefore, rather than have cysts take the place of normal tissue as occurs in the kidney, cysts in the liver seem to push aside good tissue. This appears to be the reason that normal liver function continues even with many cysts and enlarged liver size.

Liver cysts occur as often in men as in women. However, women have liver cysts at a younger age than men. Women also have more and larger cysts than men. Women who have been pregnant are more likely to have liver cysts; and the cysts are more numerous and larger in women who have been pregnant compared to women who have not been pregnant. This suggests that female hormones may influence the development of liver cysts. For this reason researchers are looking at the effect of estrogen in post-menopausal ADPKD women. Because estrogen may be a factor in liver cyst growth, the benefits of estrogen replacement therapy and the risk of increased liver cyst size must be weighed. Estrogen replacement therapy is protective against osteoporosis and heart disease. Estrogen replacement therapy also decreases vasomotor instability, which is a cause of hot flashes in post-menopausal women. Conversely, increases in the size of the liver may cause discomfort, pain and changes in appearance.

Women with ADPKD who decide to take estrogen after menopause should have an ultrasound of their liver before they start and each year or two while on their estrogen replacement therapy. This will help to evaluate if liver cysts are increasing in number and/or size. It is unclear at this time if it is better to take estrogen replacement therapy in pill form or by skin patch. More research must be done in the area of liver cysts and the role of estrogen so that we can better understand this important issue.

There have been reports of cysts in the liver becoming infected. The symptoms of liver cyst infection are fever and pain in the abdomen on the upper right side. These symptoms need to be reported to your doctor. Treatment of an infected liver cyst usually requires drainage and antibiotic therapy.

Although not common, if the liver becomes very enlarged and pain is disabling, decompression of cysts may be indicated. When there are a few large cysts, they can be drained by inserting a needle through the skin. With more cysts and greater liver involvement, a surgical procedure can be performed to unroof the cysts and/or take a section of the liver itself out. This is a major procedure that is rarely required. If needed, surgery should be done by a physician skilled in the procedure since it can be accompanied by complications.

Mitral Valve Prolapse (MVP)

Mitral valve prolapse (MVP) is a condition where the valve separating the top and the bottom of the left side of the heart does not close properly. Sometimes this causes blood to leak back to the top part of the heart. This is called regurgitation and can be heard during an examination of the heart as a heart murmur.

MVP occurs in approximately 26 percent of the people who have ADPKD compared to 2 percent to 3 percent of the general population. The majority of people with MVP never experience any major problems.

Symptoms that can be associated with MVP are palpitations, a feeling that the heart is running away or that there are extra beats in the heart, and chest pain that is not associated with exercise or exertion.

MVP is usually confirmed with an ultrasound of the heart valves called an echocardiogram. If MVP is present and causing palpitations that are bothersome, they can be treated with medications that can also treat high blood pressure at the same time. Stopping the use of caffeine, alcohol and cigarettes may be enough to decrease or stop the palpitations in many cases.

Rarely, an infection of a heart valve can occur as a complication of MVP. Although not a common occurrence, it can lead to destruction of the heart valve. Therefore, if you have MVP and a heart murmur, inform physicians who care for you. To protect your heart valve from infection, antibiotics prior to certain surgical or dental procedures may be prescribed.

Intracranial Aneurysms

An aneurysm is an outpouching in a blood vessel. Intracranial aneurysms occur in the blood vessels of the brain (figure 12). Aneurysms can leak or rupture. In these events the symptoms can include sudden severe headache, pain in moving the neck, nausea and vomiting, difficulties with speech or movement, and even loss of consciousness. All such symptoms require immediate medical attention.

Recent studies done in the United States have shown that people with ADPKD have about a 5 percent to 10 percent risk of developing intracranial aneurysms. Also, these aneurysms seem to cluster in certain families. That is, if a member of your family has an aneurysm or has ruptured an aneurysm, you may be at a higher risk of having an aneurysm, also.

Because the risk for aneurysm is small, not everyone with ADPKD needs to be tested. People who have ADPKD and a family history of aneurysm should be tested. Those whose job or hobbies would put them or others at risk if they lost consciousness (such as those who fly airplanes or drive busses) should probably be tested for aneurysms, also. It's important to inform your physician if you have a family history of intra-cranial aneurysms and/or if you have a high risk occupation or hobby.

Figure 12

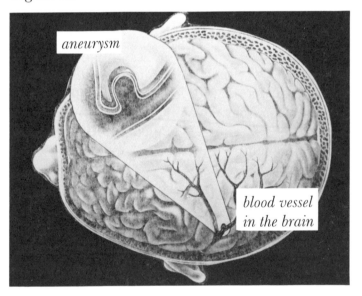

Blood vessels in the brain with an aneurysm.

High resolution CAT SCAN or MAGNETIC RESONANCE ARTERIOGRAPHY (MRA) are usually the first tests done to screen for cerebral aneurysm. If someone is allergic to dye or has decreased kidney function, an MRA is used. Both of these tests are relatively noninvasive.

If there are any areas suspicious for an aneurysm, a cerebral arteriogram is usually performed. This test is more invasive and is done by putting dye directly into the blood vessels. An arteriogram will more clearly show if there is an aneurysm and how large it is.

If an aneurysm is found in someone with ADPKD, surgical repair may be recommended. When and if surgery is performed depends on where the aneurysm is located and how large it is. Many times an aneurysm can be repaired surgically before it leaks or ruptures. People with ADPKD who have had one aneurysm may develop others over time and need close follow-up, which includes having very good control of their blood pressure.

Hernias

Both inguinal and umbilical hernias are more common in those with ADPKD. Inguinal hernias are outpouchings in the area of the groin and umbilical hernias are outpouchings at or near the navel.

Hernias should be surgically repaired if they are large or are causing other problems, just as they would be in someone who does not have ADPKD.

Diverticula

Diverticula are outpouchings on the large intestine (colon). It seems that people with ADPKD who are on dialysis or have had a transplant have diverticula more often and more complications from diverticula, including infection, than people who have other kidney diseases. At the present time we are not recommending any routine evaluation for this possible manifestation.

Pregnancy: Can I Safely Have Children if I Have ADPKD?

The diagnosis of ADPKD is no longer made many years after a person has had a family. The use of noninvasive ultrasonography has made the testing for ADPKD safe for all age groups. Thus, screening specifically for ADPKD or finding evidence of ADPKD while doing an ultrasound for other reasons has made early diagnosis a more common occurrence. Because of the earlier age of diagnosis, an understanding of the risks of pregnancy in women with ADPKD is important.

The fertility rates of both men and women who have ADPKD are no different than they are for the general population. With end-stage renal disease and dialysis, however, there is a loss of both libido and fertility. But, with a transplant, the libido most often returns to what it was prior to the loss of kidney function. Although most women do not get pregnant while on dialysis, they are not sterile.

Generally, women with ADPKD who have normal blood pressure and normal kidney function have uneventful pregnancies and deliver healthy babies. The problems associated with pregnancy and ADPKD seem to focus on increased blood pressure. Some women with ADPKD will develop new onset hypertension during their pregnancy. These women are more likely to have continued elevations in their blood pressure after delivery. Women who have high blood pressure prior to becoming pregnant have the risk of further elevations in their blood pressure while pregnant. Women who have complications in their first pregnancy are more likely to have complications in future pregnancies.

It is important for a woman with ADPKD to be closely monitored during pregnancy whether she has hypertension or not. Increases in blood pressure as well as protein in the urine could herald a serious complication in pregnancy called pre-eclampsia.

Pregnancy does not seem to affect the growth of cysts in the kidney. But there appears to be a mild long-term loss of kidney function in women who have hypertension and have four or more pregnancies, compared to ADPKD women with hypertension who have fewer than four pregnancies.

The decision to have children is a very personal one. Both the husband and wife need to discuss the risks involved and the joys associated with having a child. With an affected parent, there is a 50 percent probability of having a child who has inherited the gene for ADPKD (see genetics). Now that it is possible to determine the gene status of a fetus by gene linkage (to a 99 percent probability), attitudes on termination of pregnancy also need to be addressed.

Is There a Special Diet That Will Make My Kidneys Better or Keep Them from Getting Worse?

At this time there is no specific diet that will make polycystic kidneys better or keep them from getting worse. However, one of the functions of the kidney is to remove waste products from the body. The major source of these waste products is the food we eat, especially protein. When a great deal of kidney function is lost, these waste products back up in the blood and cause the symptoms of kidney failure. Therefore, when a person has lost a significant amount of kidney function, a low protein diet may be ordered by his/her physician.

Some studies done on both animals and humans have shown that eating large amounts of protein at one time may cause kidney function to become worse more rapidly than eating smaller amounts of protein. The recent Modification in Diet in Renal Disease (MDRD) study done by the National Institutes of Health on protein intake and kidney function did not show any benefit from lowering protein intake in individuals with ADPKD. However, the people studied already had a significant loss of kidney function.

Should I stop eating salt? High blood pressure in ADPKD does not seem to be caused by salt intake. However, excessive amounts of salt should be avoided. This becomes important when people are on certain types of blood pressure medicine and when they have kidney failure.

Can I drink alcohol? Light and/or occasional use of alcohol has not been shown to damage kidneys or the liver. However, drinking three or more ounces of alcohol a day has been associated with increases in blood pressure and can damage the liver.

Should I take extra vitamins to make sure that I'm getting all the nutrients I need? A person who eats a fairly regular diet usually does not need extra vitamins. Unlike food, vitamins are needed only in tiny amounts. Excess amounts of vitamins A, D and E can accumulate in the body and cause medical problems. Generally, if you feel you need extra vitamins, a one-a-day generic brand of vitamin is sufficient. Consult your physician before taking extra vitamins of any kind. Because there is an increased incidence of calcium kidney stones in individuals with ADPKD, women with ADPKD should discuss taking calcium supplements with their physician before they take additional calcium.

How much fluid should I drink each day? The body is usually very efficient in regulating the amount of fluid you need each day. You should drink when you are thirsty. Although the kidneys of people with ADPKD may not reabsorb fluid as efficiently as those without ADPKD, thirst is still the best way to tell how much fluid to drink.

Will caffeine damage my kidneys? There is no direct evidence that caffeine damages kidneys in people with ADPKD. However, studies done in test tubes combining ADPKD kidney cysts and caffeine-like substances have resulted in cyst growth. There is no clear relationship between caffeine and cysts in people since our bodies do not need caffeine, (some may not agree with this, especially in the morning), it may be best to limit caffeine intake to 200-250 mg a day.

CAFFEINE CONTENT OF BEVERAGES

Beverages:	Serving Size	Caffeine (mg)
Coffee, drip	5 oz	110-250
Coffee, perk	5 oz	60-125
Coffee, instant	5 oz	40-105
Coffee, decaf	5 oz	2-5
Tea, 5-minute steep	5 oz	40-100
Tea, 3-minute steep	5 oz	20-50
Hot cocoa	5 oz	2-10
Coca-cola	2 oz	45

Foods High in Potassium

Potassium is found in most foods since potassium is essential to all living cells. Legumes, whole grains, fruits, green vegetables, potatoes, meats, milk and yogurt all supply dietary potassium.

It is not wise to take potassium supplements in pill or liquid form without consulting your physician.

Can Children Also Have ADPKD?

It was once thought that people who inherited the gene for ADPKD did not form cysts or have symptoms until well into adult life. We now know that ADPKD can be diagnosed at a very young age and even in utero. If a family is informative for gene linkage, amniocentesis or chronic villous sampling can be done early in pregnancy to determine the likely gene status of the fetus. If this test is done, it must be done in conjunction with counseling so that the results of the test can be completely understood. For example, knowing that a fetus carries the ADPKD gene does not predict the course of the disease. The fetus could go on to develop ADPKD in childhood or never have a symptom until later in life.

There seem to be two different groups of children with ADPKD: those who are diagnosed in utero or in the first year of life with large kidneys and/or cysts, and those who are diagnosed after age 1.

The children who are diagnosed in the first year of life have some special characteristics. Their affected parent is most often the mother. Many times these children have brothers and/or sisters who are also diagnosed in the first year of life. Most of the children who are diagnosed in utero have large kidneys, but often they do not have actual cysts. The majority of these children develop high blood pressure in childhood, so this should be watched for and treated.

Children who are diagnosed after 1 year of age are just as likely to have an affected father as an affected mother. Often their kidneys are not large but they do have cysts. In about half the children there are only a few cysts, and in some children there may be only one cyst. In an adult one cyst is not enough to diagnose ADPKD because, as people get older, they often will develop a few kidney cysts without having ADPKD. But in children in an ADPKD family, even one cyst means they are likely to have ADPKD.

The number of cysts a child has can affect his/her signs and symptoms. Just as adults, children with many cysts are more likely to have back, side or stomach pain and are more likely to have high blood pressure than children with only a few cysts.

Almost all children who are diagnosed after the first year of life have perfectly normal kidney function that seems to stay normal throughout childhood. Although there are no studies that have followed these children into adult life, it is likely that they will maintain normal kidney function late into adult life.

What Kind of Medical Treatment Should a Child with ADPKD Have?

As with adults with ADPKD, blood pressure should be measured regularly (at least every six months) in children with ADPKD. In children, normal blood pressure is different for different ages. It is also different between boys and girls. All PKD children who are clearly hypertensive require treatment and should be seen by a children's kidney specialist (pediatric nephrologist).

Although less common than in adults, signs and symptoms of infection, blood in the urine and/or pain also need to be evaluated by a physician.

Should I Limit the Physical Activity of a Child Who Has ADPKD?

There is no information to support limiting physical activity in any child simply because he or she has ADPKD. It is possible that children with large kidneys and/or large cysts may have more episodes of blood in the urine if they play contact sports such as football. However, each child should be evaluated individually.

Should I Tell My Children They Have or Are at Risk for ADPKD?

To date, no research has been done on the effect such knowledge would have on children. Generally speaking, there is no need to burden children with information they are too young to understand. Children have a tendency to ask questions when situations arise. At that time, children usually want simple honest answers. There is no need to go into great detail unless a child asks more questions on the subject.

If parents are considering testing their children for ADPKD, the children should participate in the decision to be tested to the extent their age permits. As children get older and enter reproductive age and/or consider marriage, they should be well-informed about ADPKD.

Do Children with ADPKD Have Involvement of Organs Besides the Kidney?

Children do have some of the other nonkidney manifestations of ADPKD. Just as in adults, children who have ADPKD are more likely to have mitral valve prolapse (MVP) than children without ADPKD. Approximately 12 percent of ADPKD children will have MVP, but unlike adults it is unusual for them to have any symptoms. ADPKD children are also more likely to have hernias than children without ADPKD. When they do have hernias, they should be treated as they would in any other child. Children rarely have any of the other manifestations of ADPKD.

What Should I Do to Better Take Care of Myself if I Have ADPKD?

1.   Find a doctor who you trust and with whom you work well.

2.   Be your own expert by finding out all you can about ADPKD and any other health problems you may have. Gather as much information as possible so that you can understand your choices and make well-informed decisions. Pay attention to symptoms and write them down. Include details such as when the symptoms started, at what time of day they occur, how long they last, what makes them better or worse. This way your physician will have a clear picture of the situation when you discuss your problem with him or her. Be involved in your own health care. Ask questions and make certain you understand your care.

3.   Know about the medications you are taking. When your doctor prescribes a drug, don't be afraid to ask questions like:
- What are the advantages of this drug?
- What are the possible side effects?
- Is it dangerous to take this drug with any foods, beverage or other medications I'm taking (including over-the-counter medications)?
- Will any other condition I have be aggravated by this drug?

- Are there alternatives to this drug (generic brand, other medication, different treatment)?

Ask your pharmacist questions regarding over-the-counter medications and your medical condition. Never take medications that were prescribed for a friend or other family member.

4. Exercise on a regular basis. It was once thought that people with kidney disease were unable to participate in an active lifestyle. Since then, many studies have shown that in kidney patients exercise may be even more important than in the general population.

Regular exercise improves stamina, decreases stress, enhances a sense of well-being and may have a beneficial effect on blood pressure. And aerobic exercise is good for heart function. People do much better on dialysis and with a transplant when they are physically fit.

Generally, people with ADPKD can do any activity they want unless they get blood in the urine or the exercise causes back, flank or abdominal pain. The exercises that are least jarring to the kidneys are walking, swimming and biking. The key is to find an activity that is comfortable for you and that you enjoy doing.

How Can I Tell if My Kidneys Have Failed?

The progression to end-stage renal failure is usually gradual for people with ADPKD.

End-stage renal disease is a condition where the kidneys can no longer remove the wastes and excess water, or balance electrolytes and acids in the blood. These imbalances will result in your not feeling as well as you are used to.

Symptoms that some people experience during this time are:
>Decreased energy
>Weakness
>Shortness of breath
>Weight loss
>Nausea and/or vomiting
>Metal taste in the mouth
>Mild to moderate depression
>Decreased ability to think problems through.

Blood tests will show that your blood urea nitrogen (BUN) and creatinine are not being eliminated by the kidneys and are building up in the blood. Blood tests may also show that your electrolytes and pH are out of balance.

It's important to keep your doctor informed of your symptoms so she/he can help you decide when it's time to start therapy.

In many centers, kidney replacement therapy is done when there is about 5 percent to 10 percent of kidney function still left. If a person waits until she/he is very sick (uremic), it will take much longer to recover and may require hospitalization.

What Options Are There for Me if My Kidneys Fail?

The types of treatment for kidney failure include hemodialysis and peritoneal dialysis.

Hemodialysis - a procedure that removes extra fluid, electrolytes and wastes using a dialysis machine. Hemodialysis can be done in three different settings.

- Home hemodialysis - dialysis that is done at home with an assistant and your own dialysis machine.

- In-center, self-care hemodialysis - dialysis done in a center with you doing as much as possible with center staff helping.

- In-center hemodialysis - dialysis that is done in a center with the staff providing all of the care.

Peritoneal dialysis - a type of dialysis that removes extra fluid, electrolytes and wastes using the lining of the abdominal cavity (peritoneum). There are two ways to do peritoneal dialysis.

- Continuous ambulatory peritoneal dialysis (CAPD) - dialysis that is done on a continuous basis with exchanges four times a day.

- Continuous cyclic peritoneal dialysis (CCPD) - dialysis that is done during the night using a machine to make the exchanges while you sleep.

The basic principle of dialysis is to have the blood flow on one side of a natural or artificial membrane while there is special fluid on the other side. The membrane permits molecules that have built up in the blood to pass into the fluid and be removed.

How Will I Choose Between These Types of Treatment?

When the time comes that you need kidney replacement therapy, your physician and the dialysis team will discuss all the options available to you in detail. Often when a person gets close to needing dialysis they take a tour of the facilities that do dialysis treatments. During that time they can talk to others on dialysis and the nursing staff to get a sense of what works best for them and their family.

Are There Other Options Besides Dialysis for Those with Kidney Failure?

Kidney transplantation is another option. With transplantation, a healthy kidney is placed in the lower abdomen and takes over the function of the failed kidneys. There are two types of transplant:

- Living related donor - when a member of your family donates a kidney.

- Cadaver donor - when a kidney comes from a donor who has recently become brain dead but whose kidneys are not damaged.

Since ADPKD is a Hereditary Disorder, Can Family Members Be Kidney Donors?

A family member can be a kidney donor if that family member does not also have ADPKD. The first step for a potential donor is to have an ultrasound of his or her kidney. Eighty-three percent to

90 percent of people at risk for inheriting ADPKD can be diagnosed with ultrasound by age 30. Gene linkage can be helpful in some families when it is not clear if the potential donor has ADPKD. If the family member doesn't have ADPKD the transplant team can continue the evaluation to make sure everything else is acceptable for the person to donate a kidney.

Will My Kidneys Be Removed Before I Have a Transplant?

Usually the kidneys are not removed before a kidney transplant is performed. However, ADPKD kidneys will be removed if there have been many infections, if there is bleeding, or if there is a tumor in the kidneys. Sometimes one or both kidneys are removed if they are so large there is no room for the new kidney, or if the person is very uncomfortable or having problems eating because of kidney size.

How Are the Costs Associated with Dialysis and Transplant Covered?

In general, Medicare covers a significant amount of the cost of dialysis and transplantation. To be eligible, a person must have earned Social Security benefits or be the spouse or dependent of someone who has. About 93 percent of those with end-stage kidney disease are eligible. Those who do not qualify may be covered by Medicaid for the indigent. The social worker on the dialysis unit will help you work through the financial issues.

For more detailed information regarding Medicare and payment of costs associated with dialysis and transplant, call your local Social Security Medicare office or write to the U.S. Department of Health and Human Services (address in back of booklet) for the Medicare Handbook. The National Kidney Foundation also has published a booklet on these issues. Another good source of information for Medicare coverage and kidney replacement therapy is your local transplant unit.

Common Tests Done When a Person Has ADPKD

BLOOD TESTS

Creatinine is a measure of kidney function. It is a waste product of muscle metabolism (the work the muscles do). After creatinine leaves the muscles, it enters into the blood, is filtered by the kidneys and ends up in the urine. So there is always some creatinine in the blood and some in the urine. When there is a loss in kidney function, the kidneys do not clear creatinine from the blood as efficiently as they once did. This causes an increase of creatinine in the blood, which can be measured.

Normal blood creatinine is 0.6 to 1.4 mg/dl. When a person's blood creatinine goes up to 2.0 mg/dl, they have lost approximately half of their kidney function.

Blood urea nitrogen (BUN) is another measure of kidney function. Urea nitrogen is the waste product of dietary protein. If there is a loss of kidney function, the urea nitrogen builds up in the blood. A number of factors such as diet, protein intake, heart function and fluid status can affect BUN. Therefore, creatinine is the measure of kidney function that is followed more regularly. The normal range for BUN is 6 to15 mg/dl.

Liver function tests are also blood tests. Liver function is almost always normal even if there are cysts in the liver. If at some time your liver function tests are not in the normal range, your physician should look for a cause other than ADPKD.

URINE TESTS

White blood cells (WBC) in urine. WBCs normally are present only in small numbers in the urine, and some people with ADPKD do pass a a few more. However, large numbers of WBCs in the urine suggest a urinary tract infection. If this happens, your doctor will culture your urine to determine if and what types of bacteria are present.

Red blood cells (RBC) in the urine. Only a few RBCs are normally found in the urine. As with white blood cells, some people with ADPKD also pass a few RBCs. Sometimes with an episode of bleeding, there are so many RBCs that they color the urine pink, red or brown (see hematuria).

Protein in the urine. Protein is normally found in the urine only in small amounts. About one-third of those with ADPKD pass protein into the urine, but it is usually less than a gram in 24 hours. If protein loss is greater than one gram in 24 hours, there may be another problem occurring in the kidney along with ADPKD.

24-hour urine collection. This test is done in combination with the blood creatinine test to determine kidney function, called creatinine clearance or glomerular filtration rate (GFR).

Imaging studies. Studies used to see or image organs or blood vessels in the body.

Ultrasonography is a test done with sound waves. Ultrasonography does not require the use of radiation or contrast dye to be injected into a person. It can be done safely in pregnant women.

Because it's so safe and accurate, ultrasonography is the most common imaging test done to screen for and follow progression of ADPKD.

Echocardiogram is an ultrasound of the heart. One of the uses of an echocardiogram is to image the valves of the heart. Your physician may order this test if he or she suspects you have mitral valve prolapse (MVP).

Computed Axial Tomography (CT Scan) is a sophisticated form of x-ray. CT scan uses radiation and, most often, contrast dye to visualize the organ or blood vessels being studied. This imaging technique is very helpful if complications of ADPKD arise, such as bleeding into a cyst or kidney stones.

High-resolution CT scan is used to visualize the blood vessels in the brain. This type of CT can show if there are any suspicious areas that may be aneurysms before doing more invasive or expensive studies.

Magnetic Resonance Imaging (MRI) takes pictures of the body using a magnet that puts a certain spin on particles that exist in a person's body. It does not require contrast dyes or radiation. Although cysts are easily visualized with MRI, it is a more expensive test and it does not appear any better than ultrasonography for diagnosing or following ADPKD.

Magnetic Resonance Arteriogram (MRA) is used to visualize the blood vessels in the brain for screening of aneurysms. This is similar to high-resolution CT, but does not use contrast dyes or radiation. MRA is used when people are allergic to contrast dyes and/or iodine, or if they have lost kidney function.

Arteriograms are procedures that utilize contrast dye injected into the blood vessels in order to clearly visualize them. When it is suspected that there is an aneurysm on a blood vessel in the brain, an arteriogram is usually done.

References:

Exercise and the Kidney Patient
National Kidney Foundation
30 East 33rd Street
New York, New York 10016

Medicare: Coverage of Kidney Dialysis and Kidney
        Transplantation Services
Medicare Handbook
U.S. Department of Health and Human Services
Health Care Financing Administration

ADPKD Review Article
Patricia A. Gabow, MD
New England Journal of Medicine
329: 332-342 (July 29), 1993

ADPKD: More Than a Kidney Disease
Patricia A. Gabow, MD
American Journal of Kidney Diseases
Volume XVI, No. 5 (Nov.)
403-413, 1990

Proceedings of the Fifth International Workshop
        on Polycystic Kidney Disease
PKR Foundation
4901 Main Street, Ste. 320
Kansas City, Missouri 64112